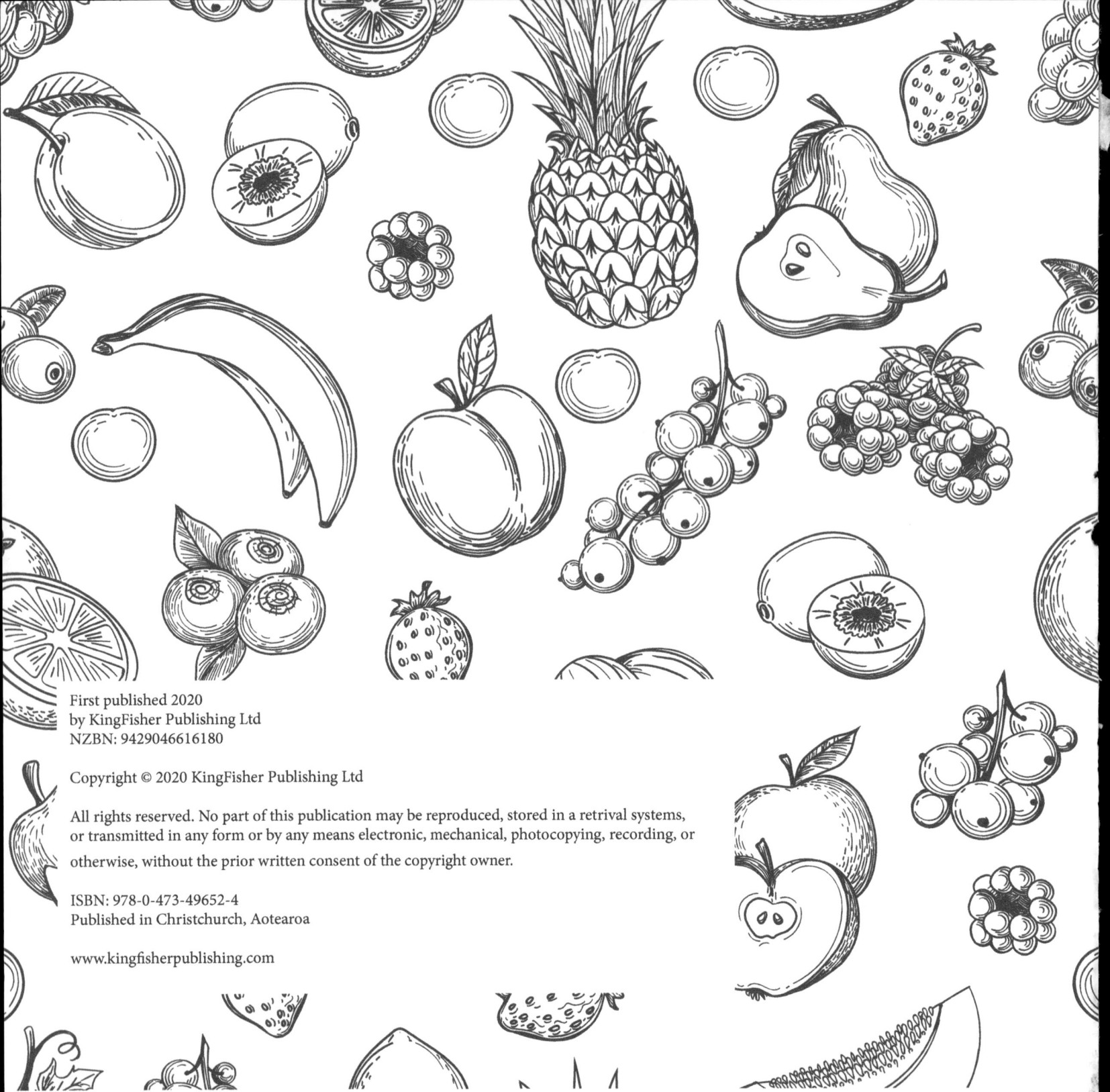

First published 2020
by KingFisher Publishing Ltd
NZBN: 9429046616180

Copyright © 2020 KingFisher Publishing Ltd

All rights reserved. No part of this publication may be reproduced, stored in a retrieval systems, or transmitted in any form or by any means electronic, mechanical, photocopying, recording, or otherwise, without the prior written consent of the copyright owner.

ISBN: 978-0-473-49652-4
Published in Christchurch, Aotearoa

www.kingfisherpublishing.com

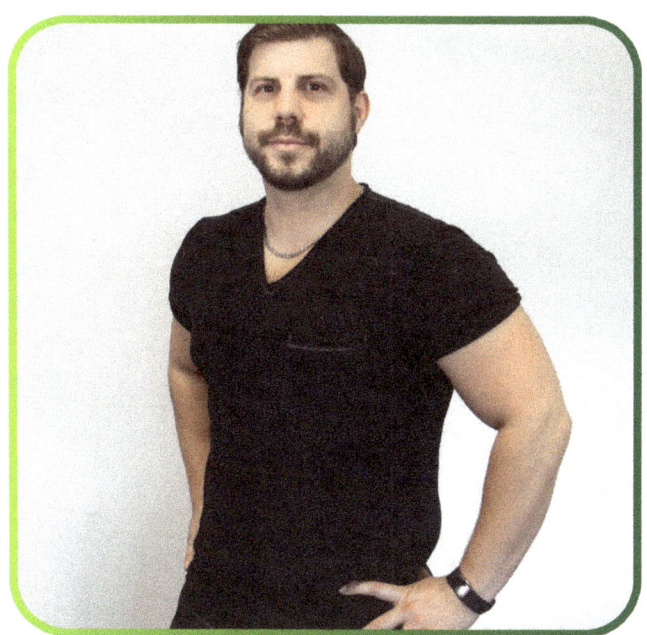

Here at Kingfisher Fitness we truly believe that good health and fitness starts in the kitchen. The purpose of our springtime smoothie book is to provide you with a quick, efficient and delicious way to eat fresh. You'll notice that our procedure for producing fantastic smoothies remains consistent. This allows for the true focus to be on the fresh, healthy ingredients and the wonderful adventure that is flavour pairing. As always good mental and physical wellbeing starts with quality nutrition.

All the best,

Ronnie Fisher

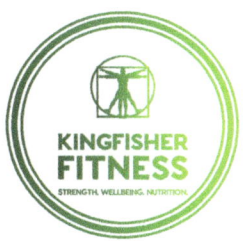

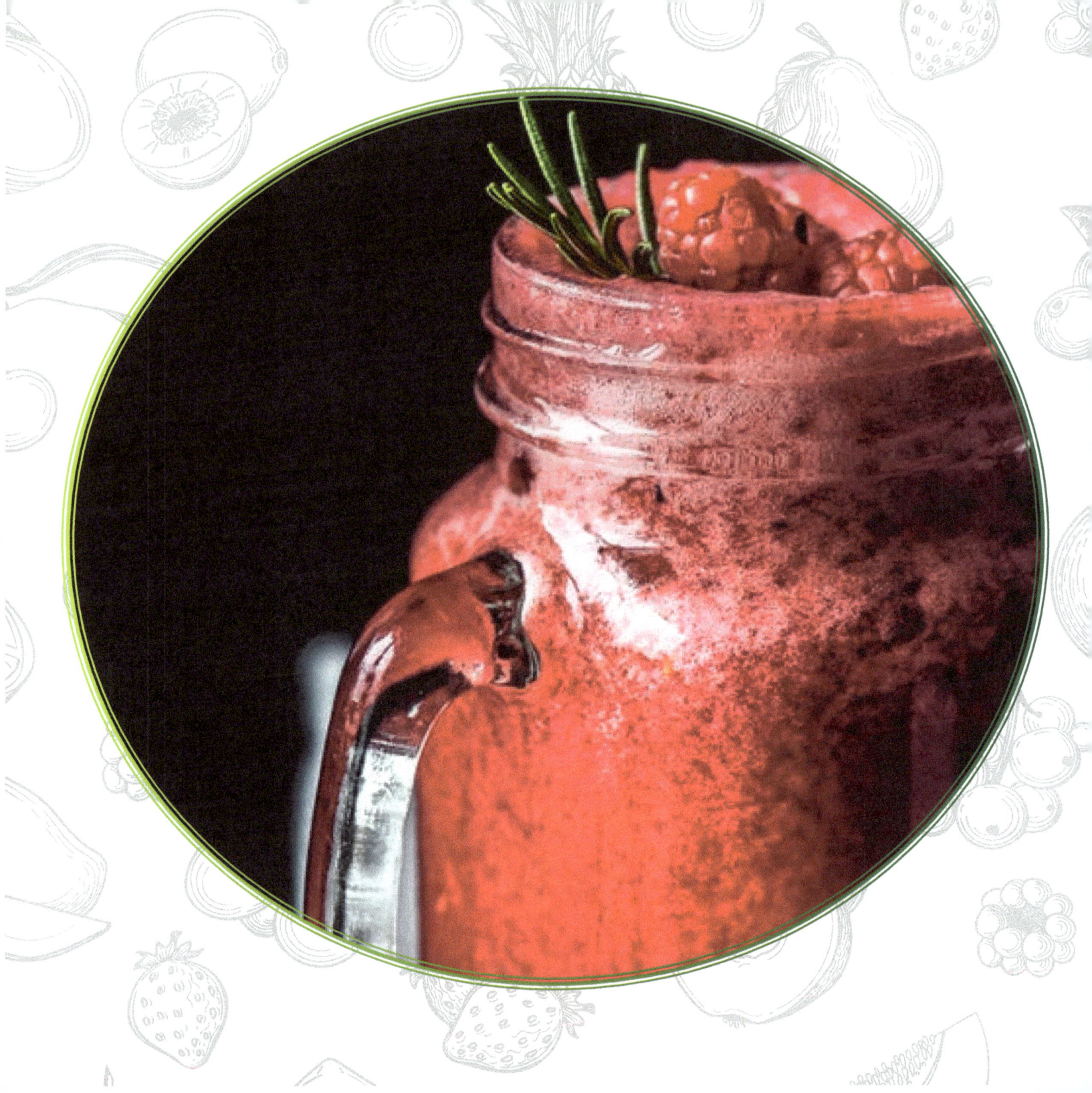

Berrynana

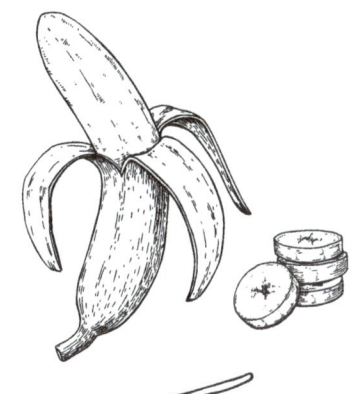

INGREDIENTS:

2 banana

1 cup strawberries

1/2 cup raspberries

1/2 cup cherrys

1 cup water

8 ice cubes

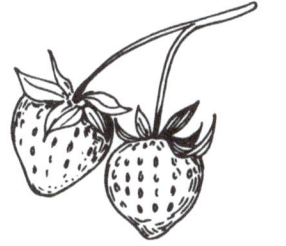

PROCEDURE:

1) Remove peels, seeds, stems and piths from all fruit before blending.

2) Place liquid into blender (water, coconut milk, almond milk can also be used) with ice cubes. Blend till ice begins to break.

3) Add solid fruit first, blend, then add softer fruit and yoghurt if required and blend till smooth.

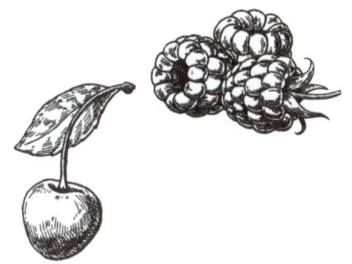

Do something today that Future You will be proud of.

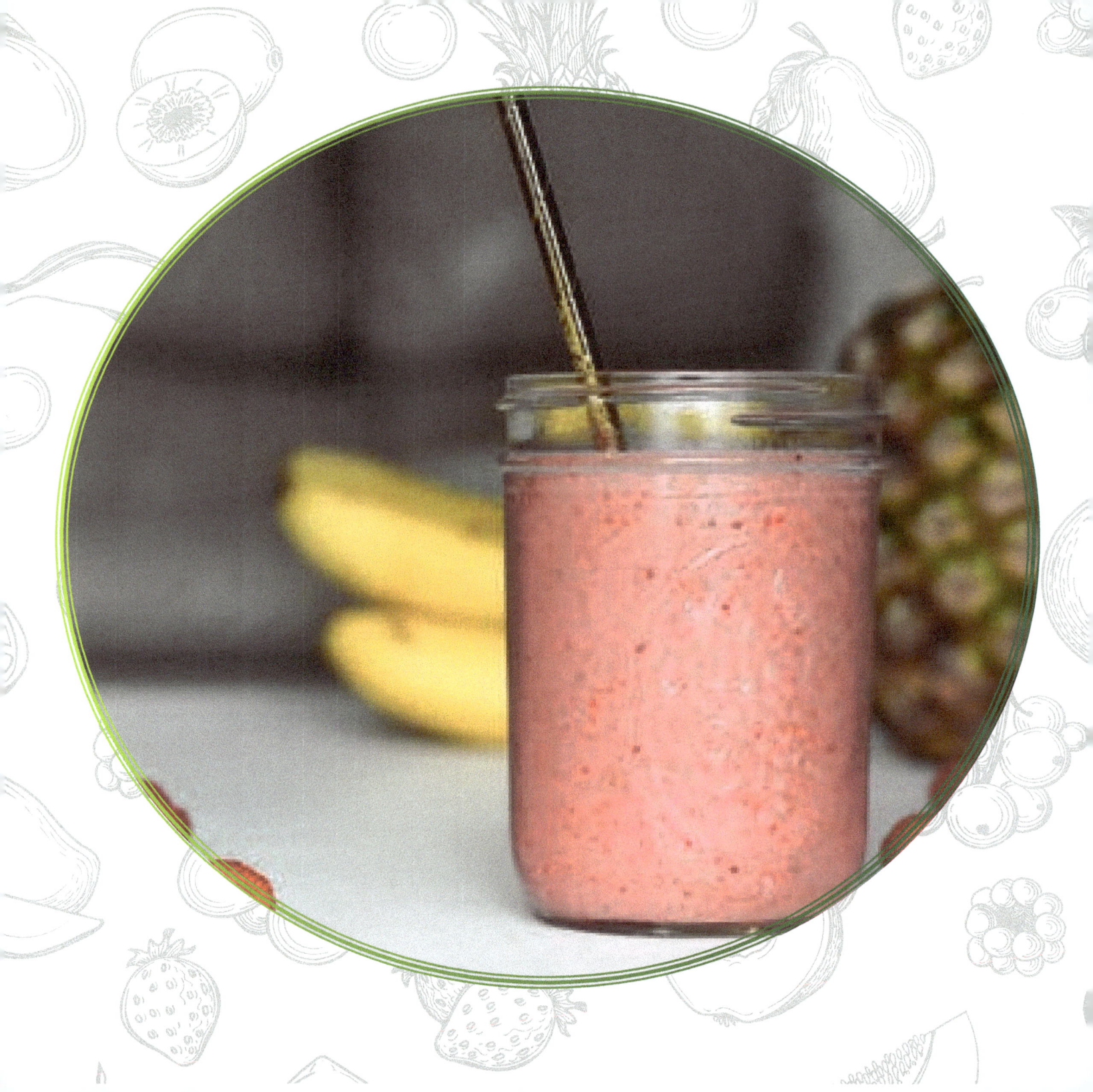

Orange & Pineapple

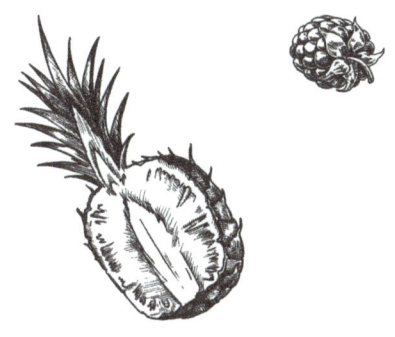

Ingredients:

1 pineapple (peeled, cored & chopped)

½ cup raspberries

Juice from 1 orange

1 banana

1 cup coconut milk

½ cup coconut yoghurt

5 ice cubes

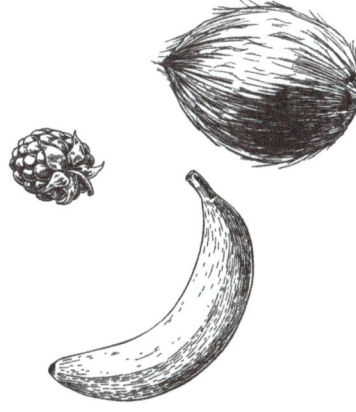

Procedure:

1) Remove peels, seeds, stems and piths from all fruit before blending.

2) Place liquid into blender (water, coconut milk, almond milk can also be used) with ice cubes. Blend till ice begins to break.

3) Add solid fruit first, blend, then add softer fruit and yoghurt if required and blend till smooth.

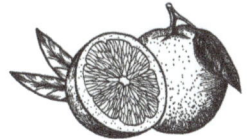

One day or Day One.
You decide.

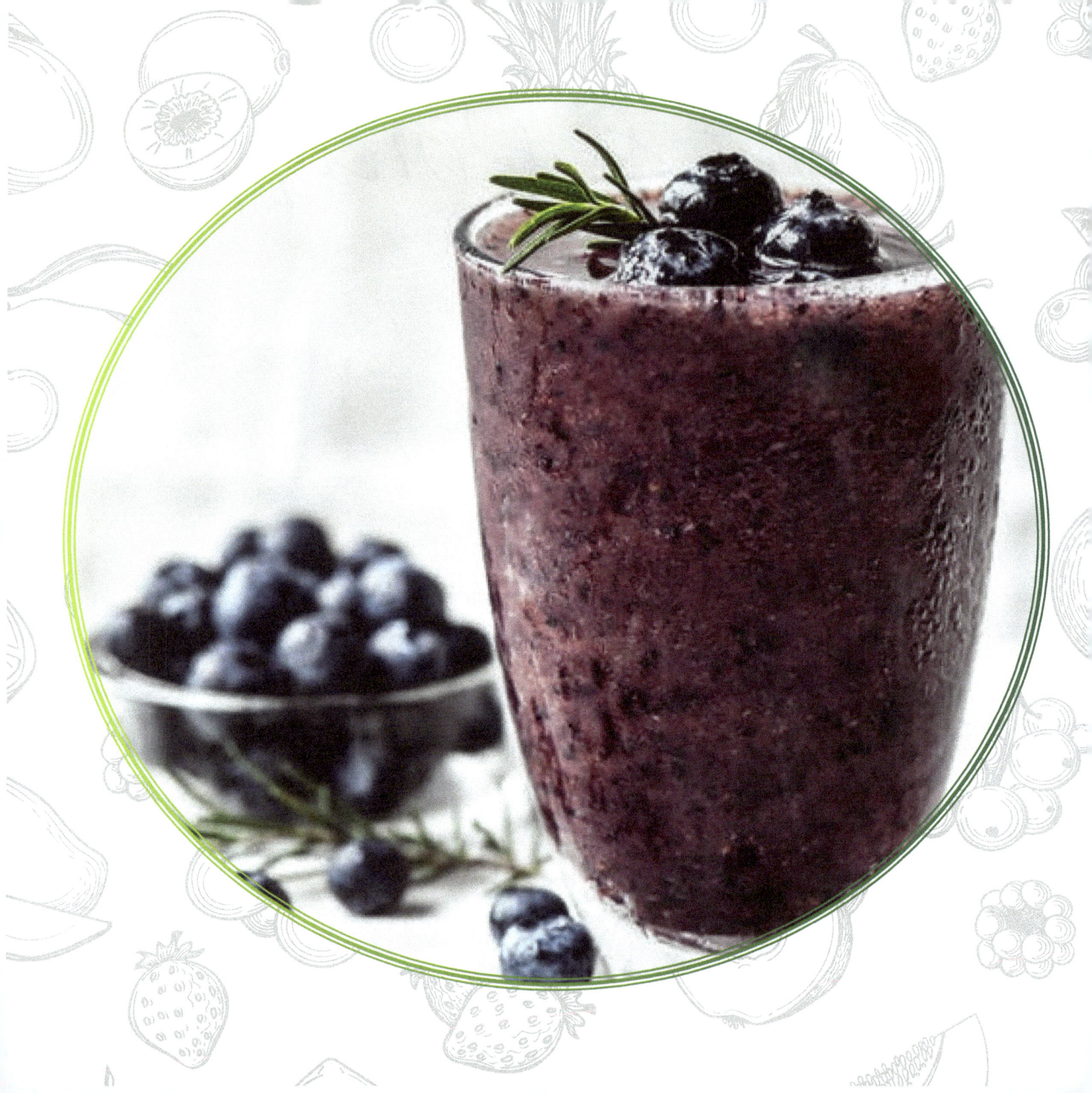

Beautiful Blueberry

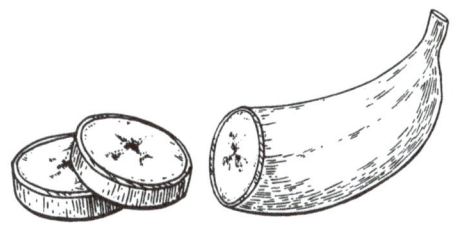

INGREDIENTS:

1 banana

2 cups blueberries

¾ cup coconut

½ cup water

4 ice cubes

½ tsp cinnamon

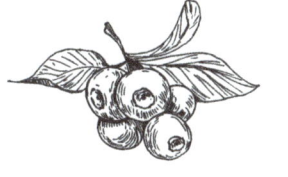

PROCEDURE:

1) Remove peels, seeds, stems and piths from all fruit before blending.

2) Place liquid into blender (water, coconut milk, almond milk can also be used) with ice cubes. Blend till ice begins to break.

3) Add solid fruit first, blend, then add softer fruit and yoghurt if required and blend till smooth.

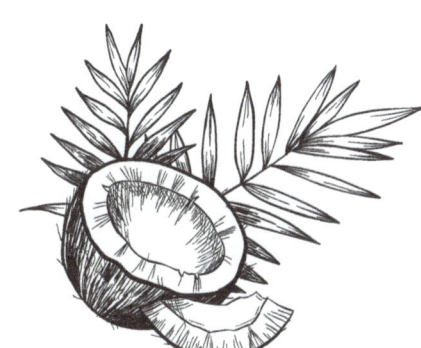

Ask yourself "is what you are doing today helping you get to where you want to be tomorrow?"

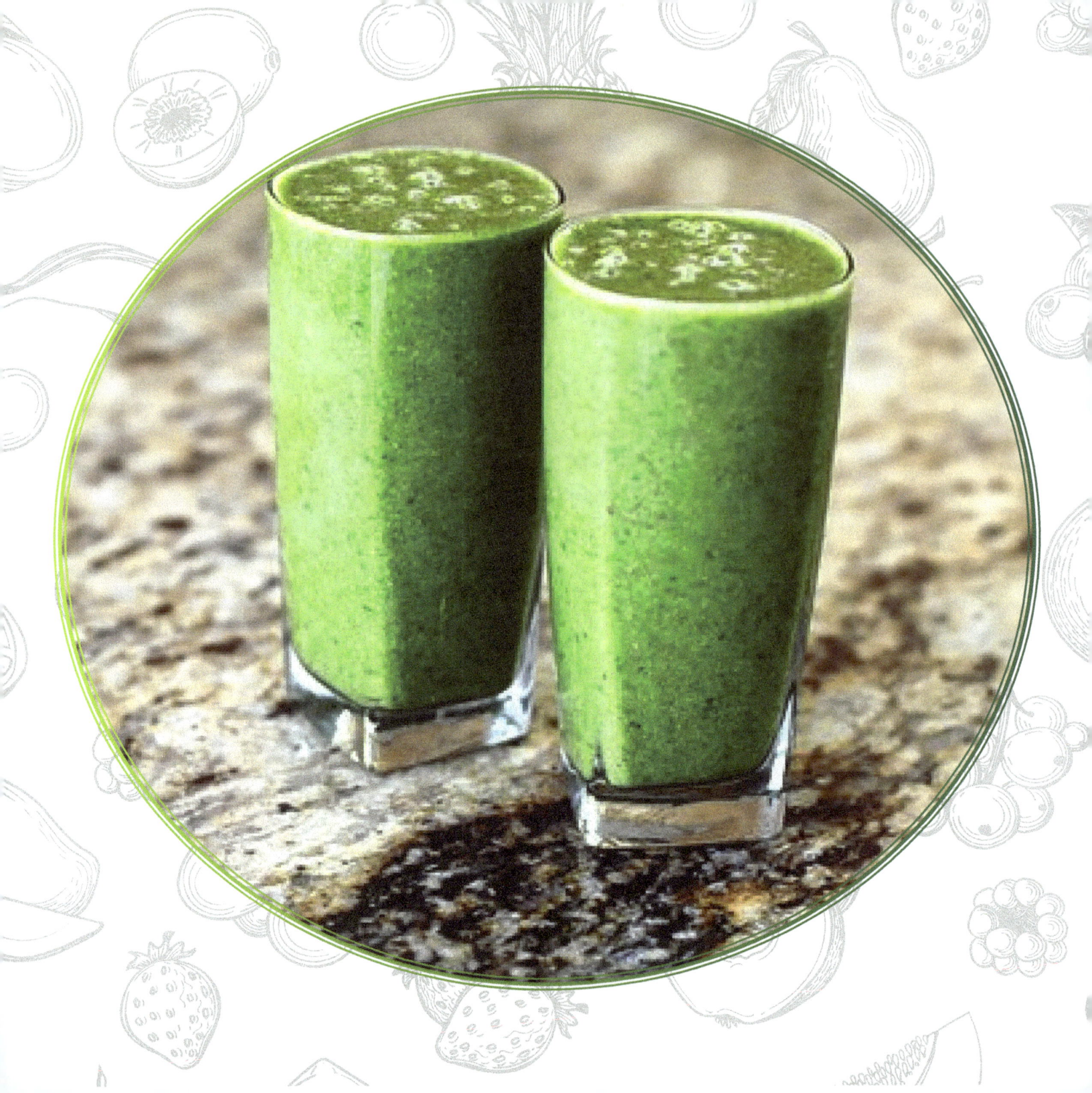

Avocado Greens

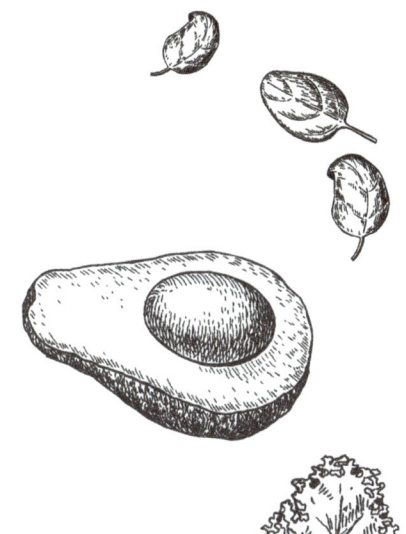

Ingredients:

1 banana

1 cup kale

1 cup spinach

2 avocado

¼ cup coconut yoghurt

1 cup coconut milk

6 ice cubes

Procedure:

1) Remove peels, seeds, stems and piths from all fruit before blending.

2) Place liquid into blender (water, coconut milk, almond milk can also be used) with ice cubes. Blend till ice begins to break.

3) Add solid fruit first, blend, then add softer fruit and yoghurt if required and blend till smooth.

There is no failure.
You either win or you learn.

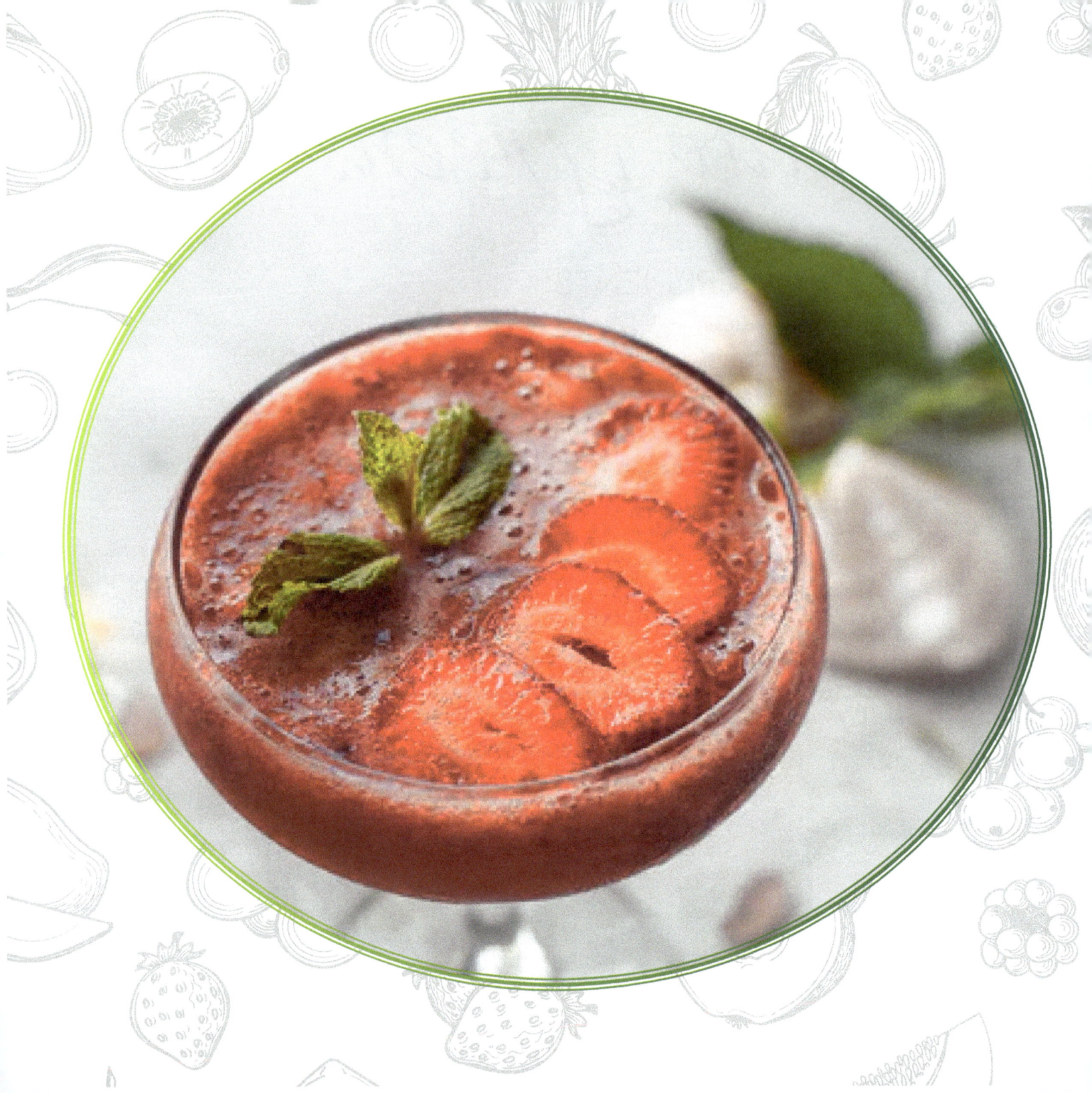

Apple Red

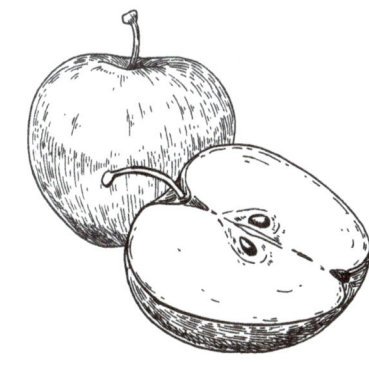

INGREDIENTS:

1 banana

1 cup cherries

2 red apples

½ cup strawberries

½ cup coconut yoghurt

1 cup coconut milk

6 ice cubes

1 tsp honey

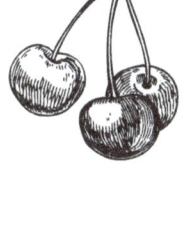

PROCEDURE:

1) Remove peels, seeds, stems and piths from all fruit before blending.

2) Place liquid into blender (water, coconut milk, almond milk can also be used) with ice cubes. Blend till ice begins to break.

3) Add solid fruit first, blend, then add softer fruit and yoghurt if required and blend till smooth.

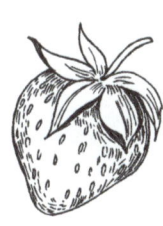

You already have what it takes.

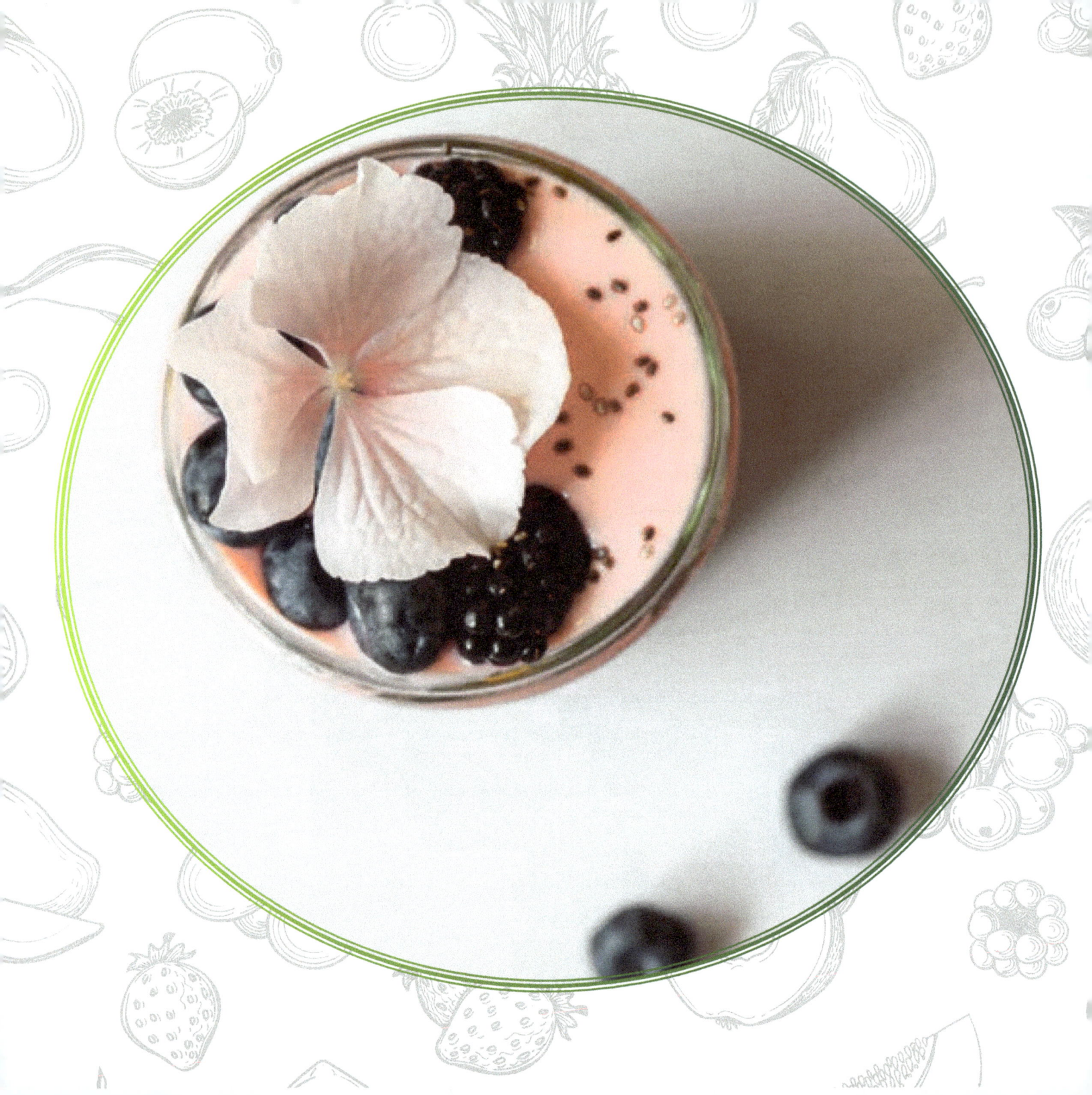

Apricot Mango

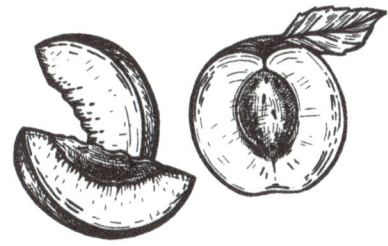

Ingredients:

5 apricots

2 mangoes

1 lemon

8 ice cubes

½ cup coconut yoghurt

¾ cup water

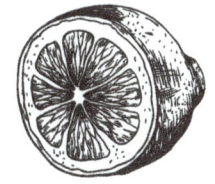

Procedure:

1) Remove peels, seeds, stems and piths from all fruit before blending.

2) Place liquid into blender (water, coconut milk, almond milk can also be used) with ice cubes. Blend till ice begins to break.

3) Add solid fruit first, blend, then add softer fruit and yoghurt if required and blend till smooth.

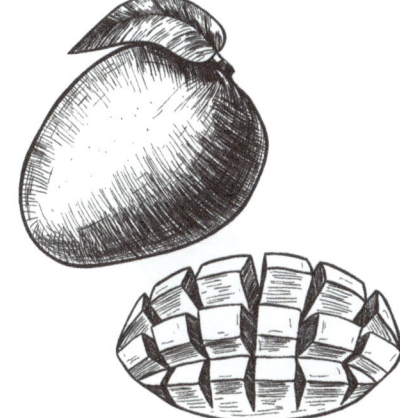

Strive for PROGRESS, not Perfection.

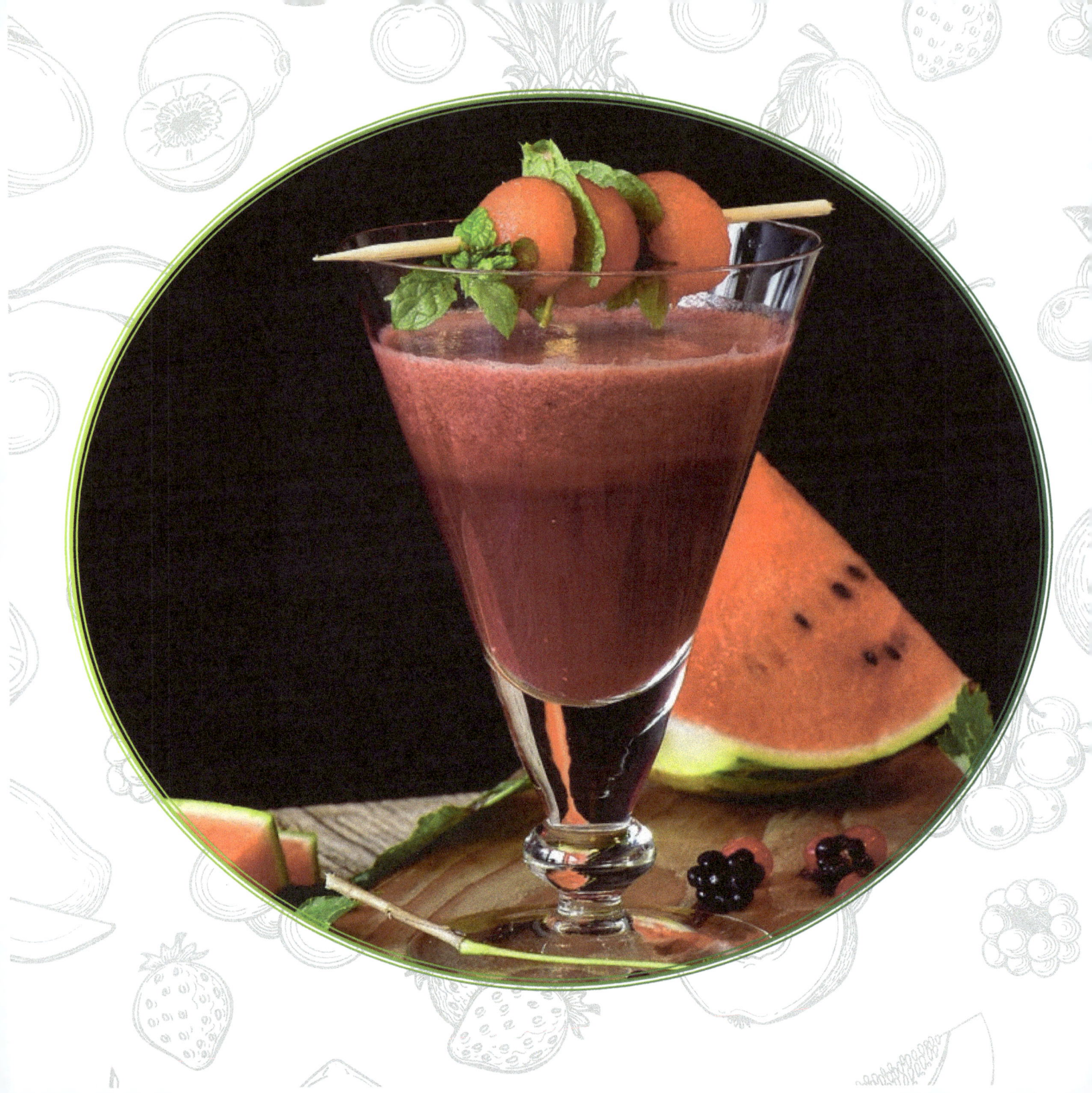

Berry Melondary

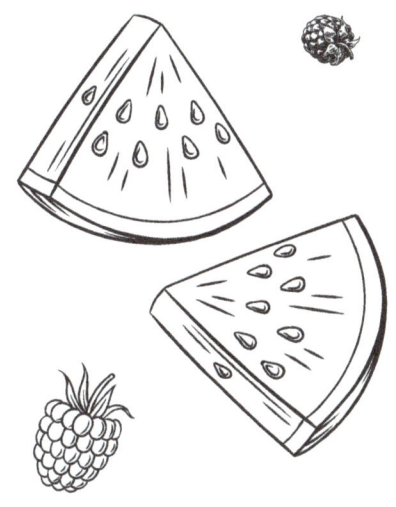

INGREDIENTS:

1 cup boysenberries

1 cup watermelon

1 cup strawberries

1 cup raspberries

1 banana

1 cup coconut milk

6 ice cubes

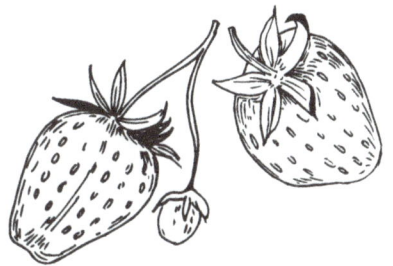

PROCEDURE:

1) Remove peels, seeds, stems and piths from all fruit before blending.

2) Place liquid into blender (water, coconut milk, almond milk can also be used) with ice cubes. Blend till ice begins to break.

3) Add solid fruit first, blend, then add softer fruit and yoghurt if required and blend till smooth.

Every breath you take with a smile, is a breath that leads to your future happiness.

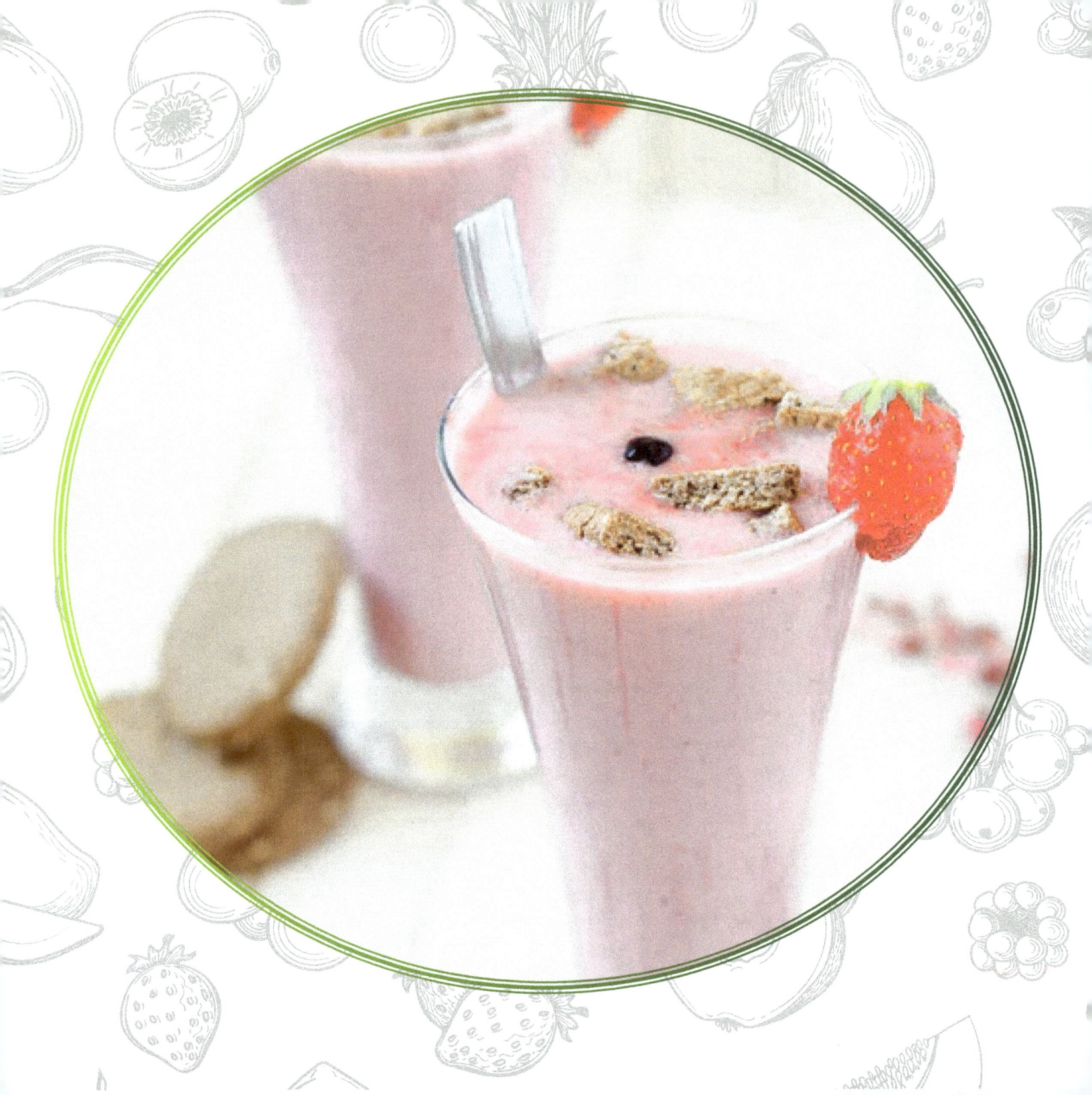

Berry Tropic

INGREDIENTS:

1 banana

1 pineapple

1/3 cup mango

1 cup strawberries

1 cup raspberries

½ cup coconut yoghurt

1 cup coconut milk

PROCEDURE:

1) Remove peels, seeds, stems and piths from all fruit before blending.

2) Place liquid into blender (water, coconut milk, almond milk can also be used) with ice cubes. Blend till ice begins to break.

3) Add solid fruit first, blend, then add softer fruit and yoghurt if required and blend till smooth.

Always believe that something WONDERFUL is about to happen.

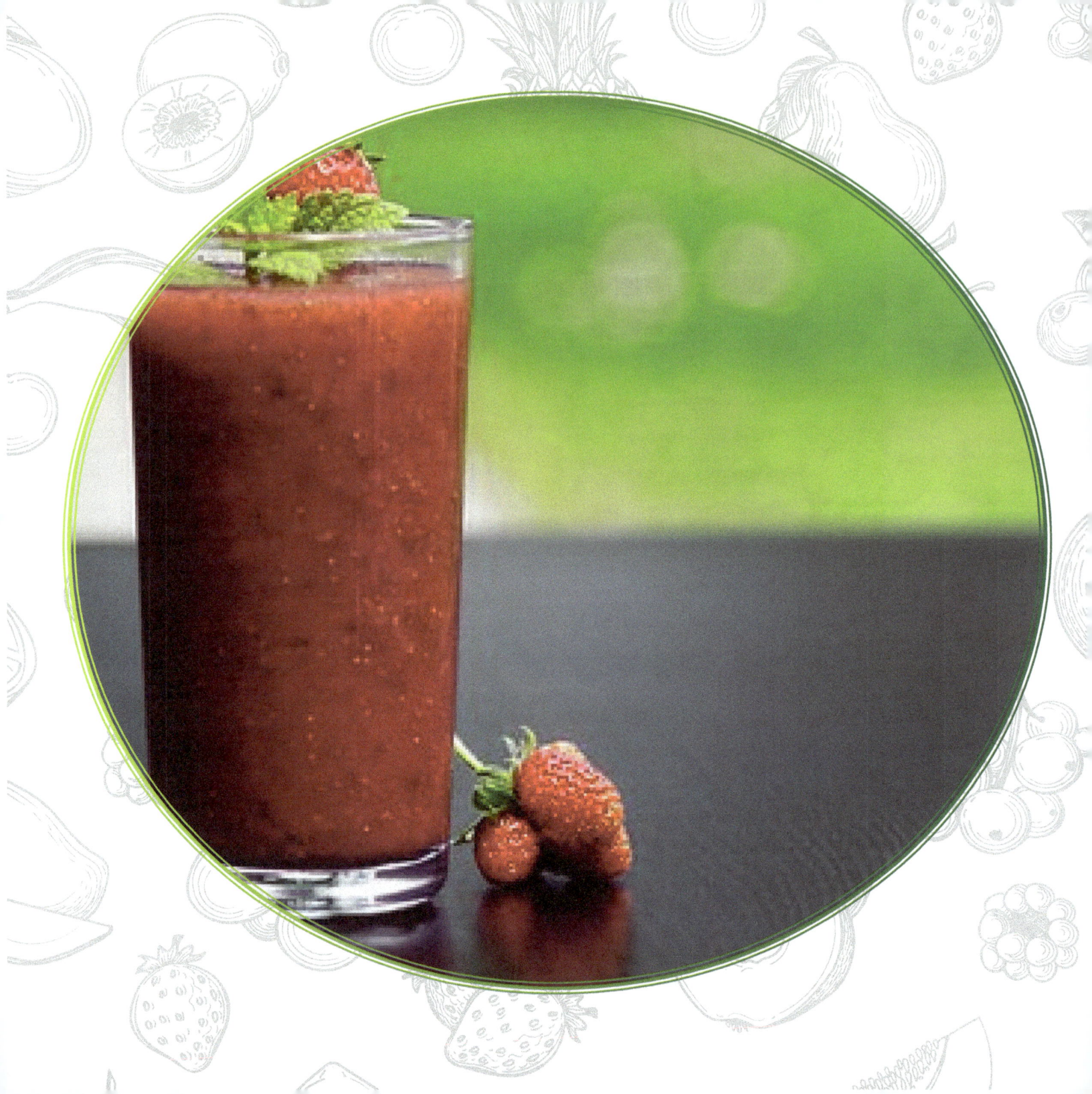

Cherry Berry Peach

Ingredients:

2 peaches

1 cup cherries

1 cup strawberries

1 banana

½ cup coconut yoghurt

1 cup coconut milk

5 ice cubes

Procedure:

1) Remove peels, seeds, stems and piths from all fruit before blending.

2) Place liquid into blender (water, coconut milk, almond milk can also be used) with ice cubes. Blend till ice begins to break.

3) Add solid fruit first, blend, then add softer fruit and yoghurt if required and blend till smooth.

Be fearless in the pursuit of what sets your soul on fire

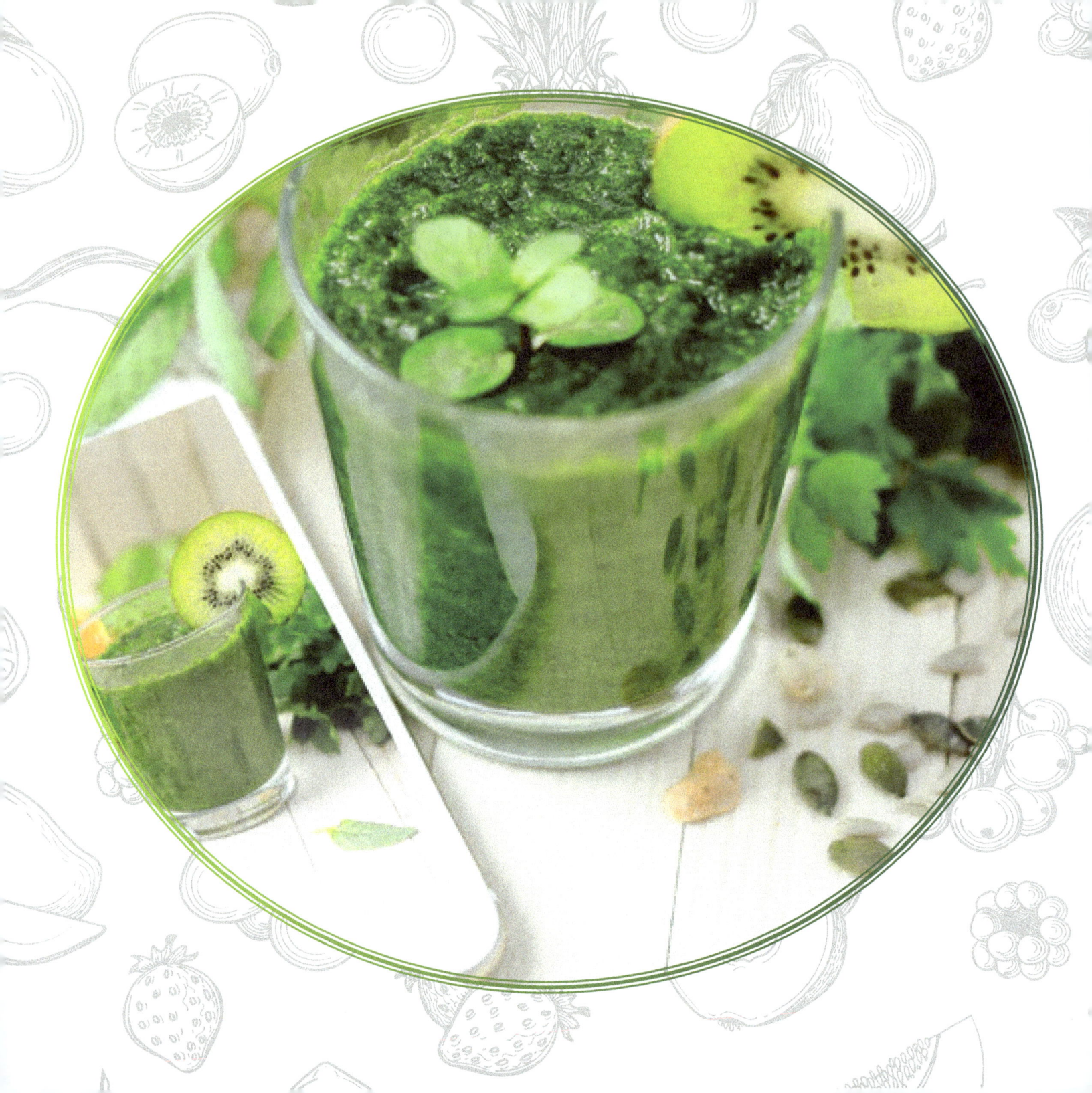

The Clean Green

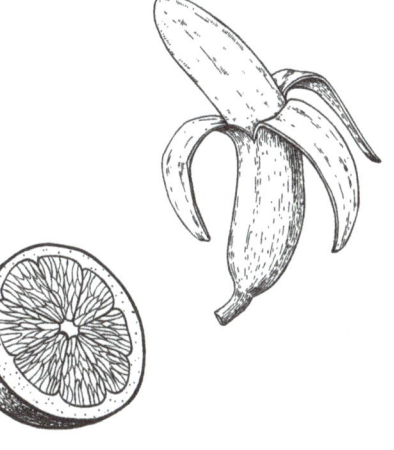

Ingredients:

1 banana

Juice from 1 orange

2 cups kale

1 cup kiwi fruit

½ cup cucumber

6 ice cubes

¾ cup water

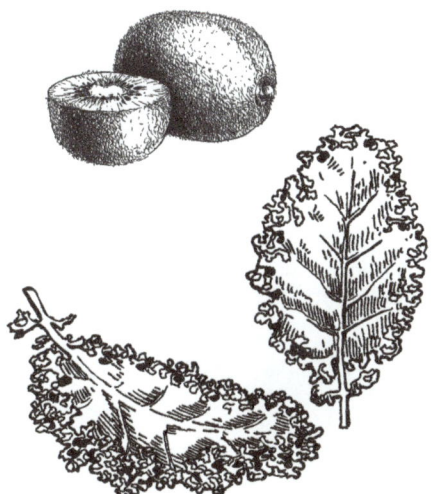

Procedure:

1) Remove peels, seeds, stems and piths from all fruit before blending.

2) Place liquid into blender (water, coconut milk, almond milk can also be used) with ice cubes. Blend till ice begins to break.

3) Add solid fruit first, blend, then add softer fruit and yoghurt if required and blend till smooth.

Walk with your head held high. You are the most beautiful being on this earth.

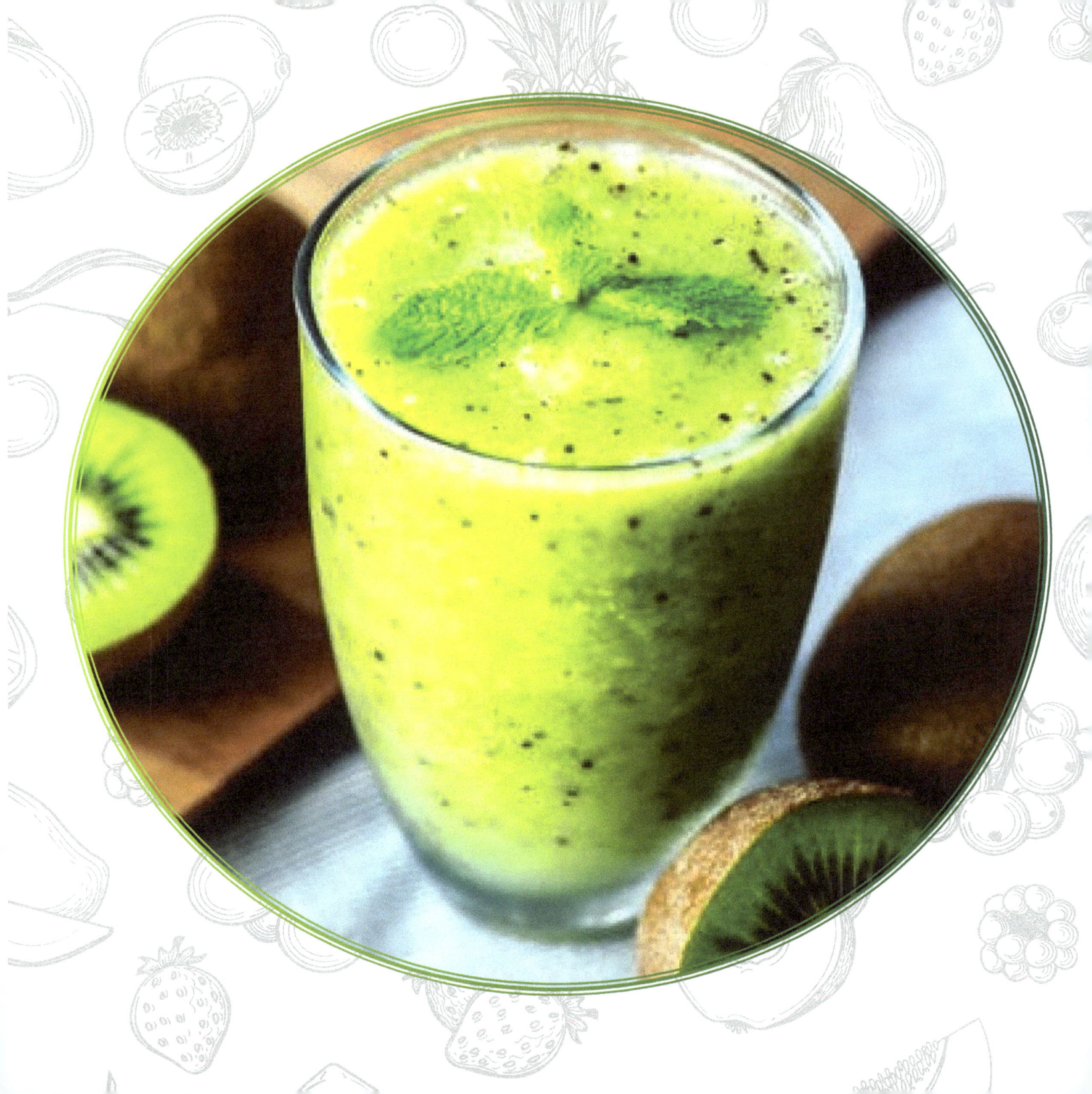

The Kiwi Green

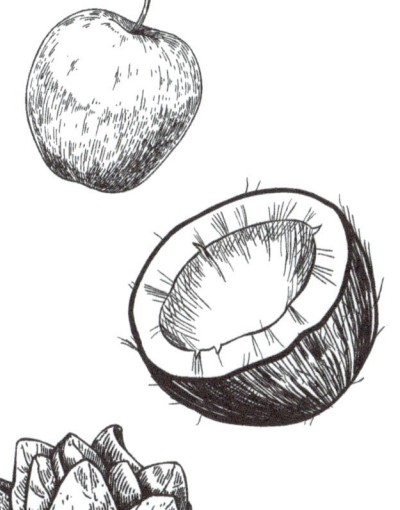

Ingredients:

1 apple Cored

3 kiwi fruit peeled

1 cup spinach

½ cup coconut yoghurt

1 cup coconut milk

1 tbsp honey

Procedure:

1) 1) Remove peels, seeds, stems and piths from all fruit before blending.

2) 2) Place liquid into blender (water, coconut milk, almond milk can also be used) with ice cubes. Blend till ice begins to break.

3) 3) Add solid fruit first, blend, then add softer fruit and yoghurt if required and blend till smooth.

Live your best life every day

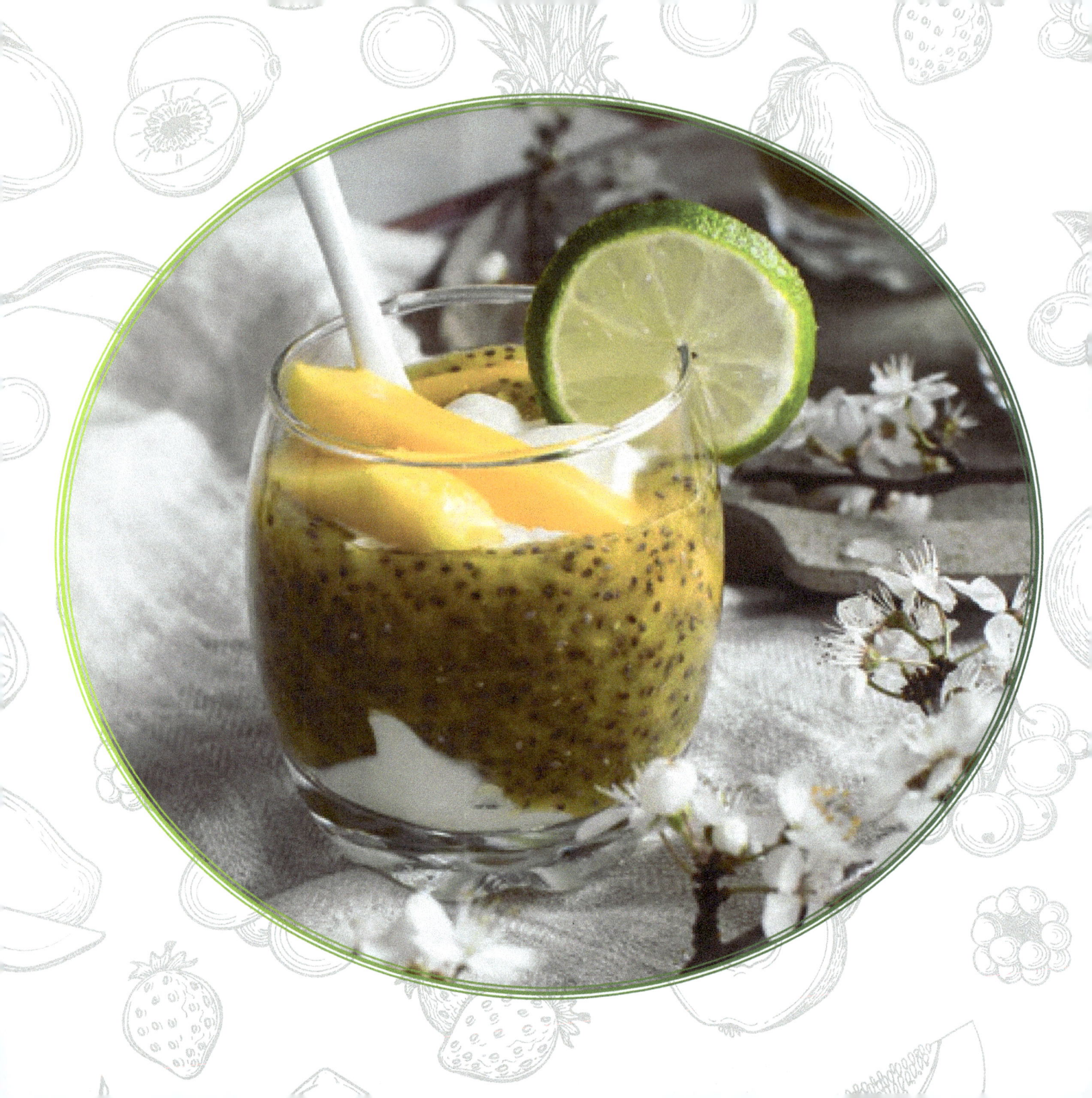

Mango Kiwi

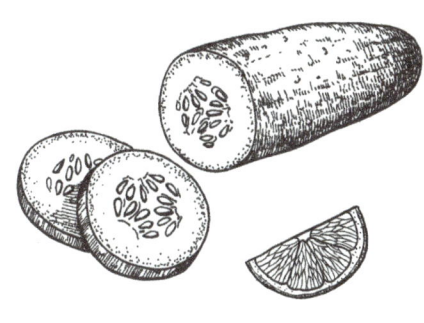

Ingredients:

1 cucumber

1 lime juiced

1 mango

3 kiwi fruit

2 pears

1/2 cup spinach

6 ice cubes

1 cup water

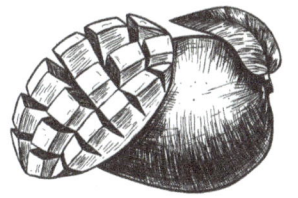

Procedure:

1) Remove peels, seeds, stems and piths from all fruit before blending.

2) Place liquid into blender (water, coconut milk, almond milk can also be used) with ice cubes. Blend till ice begins to break.

3) Add solid fruit first, blend, then add softer fruit and yoghurt if required and blend till smooth

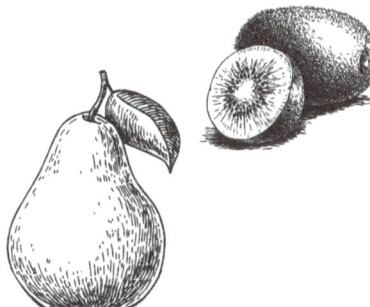

Do the small things in a great way.

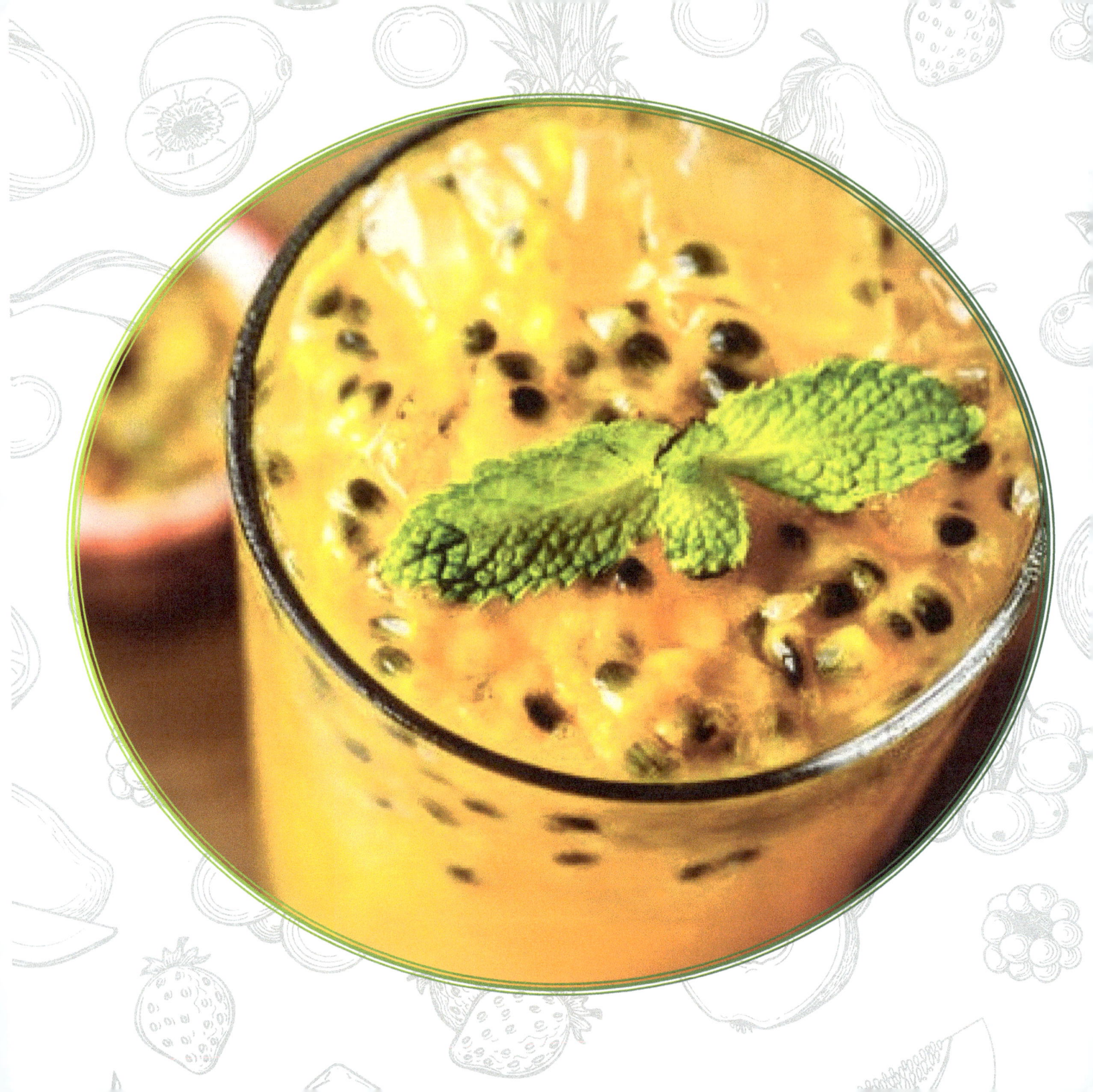

Tropical Passion

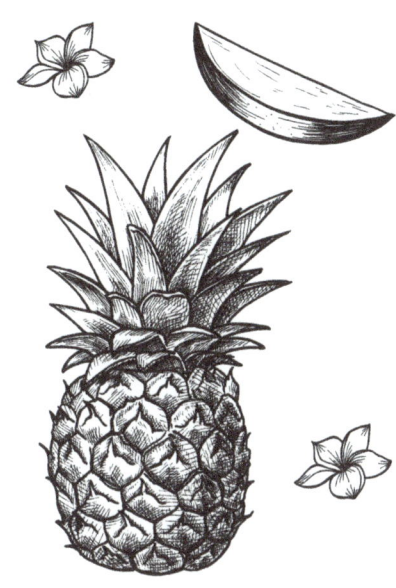

INGREDIENTS:

1 papaya

1 passionfruit

1 pineapple

1 mango

1 cup coconut milk

½ cup coconut yoghurt

6 ice cubes

1 tsp honey

PROCEDURE:

1) Remove peels, seeds, stems and piths from all fruit before blending.

2) Place liquid into blender (water, coconut milk, almond milk can also be used) with ice cubes. Blend till ice begins to break.

3) Add solid fruit first, blend, then add softer fruit and yoghurt if required and blend till smooth.

It will never be perfect. Finish it now

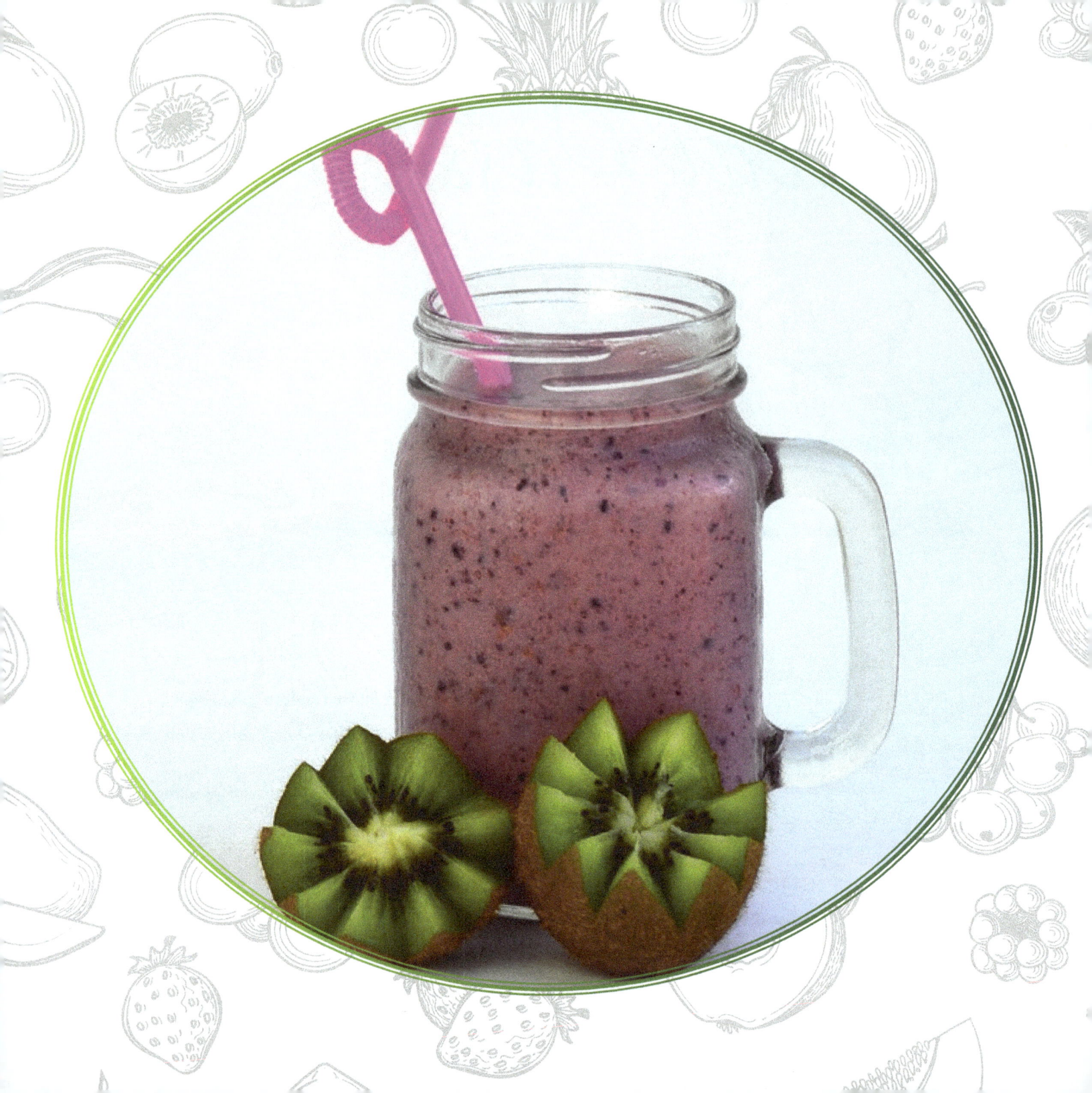

Strawberry Kiwi

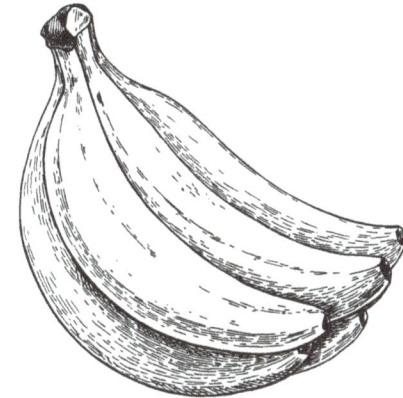

Ingredients:

1 banana

1 cup strawberries

2 kiwi fruit

1 cup coconut milk

½ cup coconut yoghurt

Procedure:

1) 1) Remove peels, seeds, stems and piths from all fruit before blending.

2) 2) Place liquid into blender (water, coconut milk, almond milk can also be used) with ice cubes. Blend till ice begins to break.

3) 3) Add solid fruit first, blend, then add softer fruit and yoghurt if required and blend till smooth.

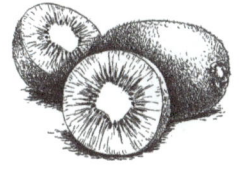

IF NOTHING EVER CHANGED, THERE WOULD BE NO BUTTERFLIES.

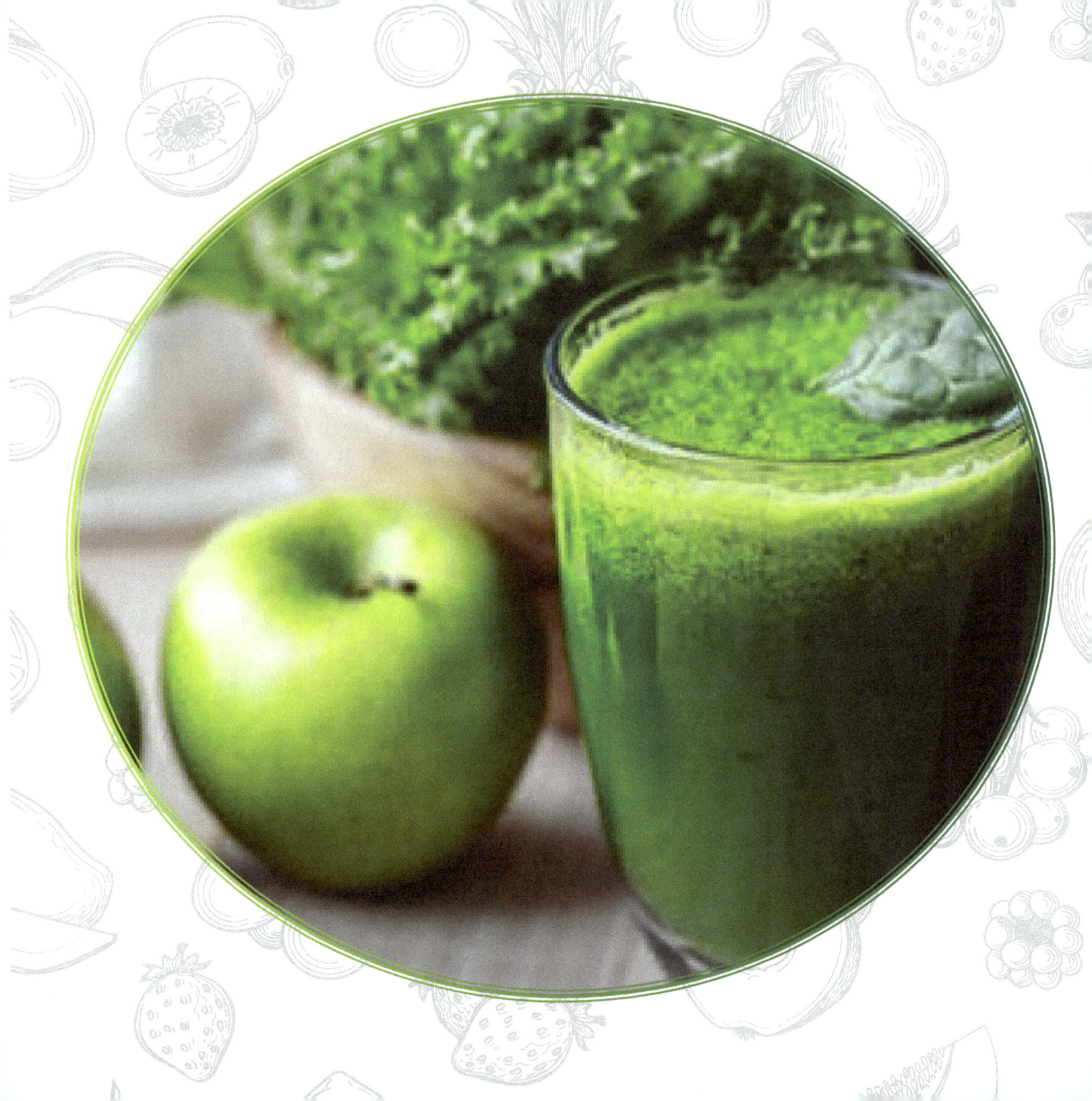

Super Green Apple

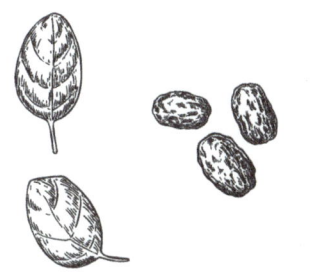

Ingredients:

1 cup spinach

1 red apple

1 green apple

2 kiwi fruit

3 dates pitted

8 ice cubes

¾ cup water

1 banana

½ tsp cinnamon

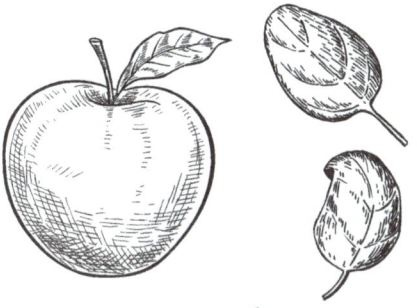

Procedure:

1) Remove peels, seeds, stems and piths from all fruit before blending.

2) Place liquid into blender (water, coconut milk, almond milk can also be used) with ice cubes. Blend till ice begins to break.

3) Add solid fruit first, blend, then add softer fruit and yoghurt if required and blend till smooth.

If you do not drive the change in your life, somebody else will.

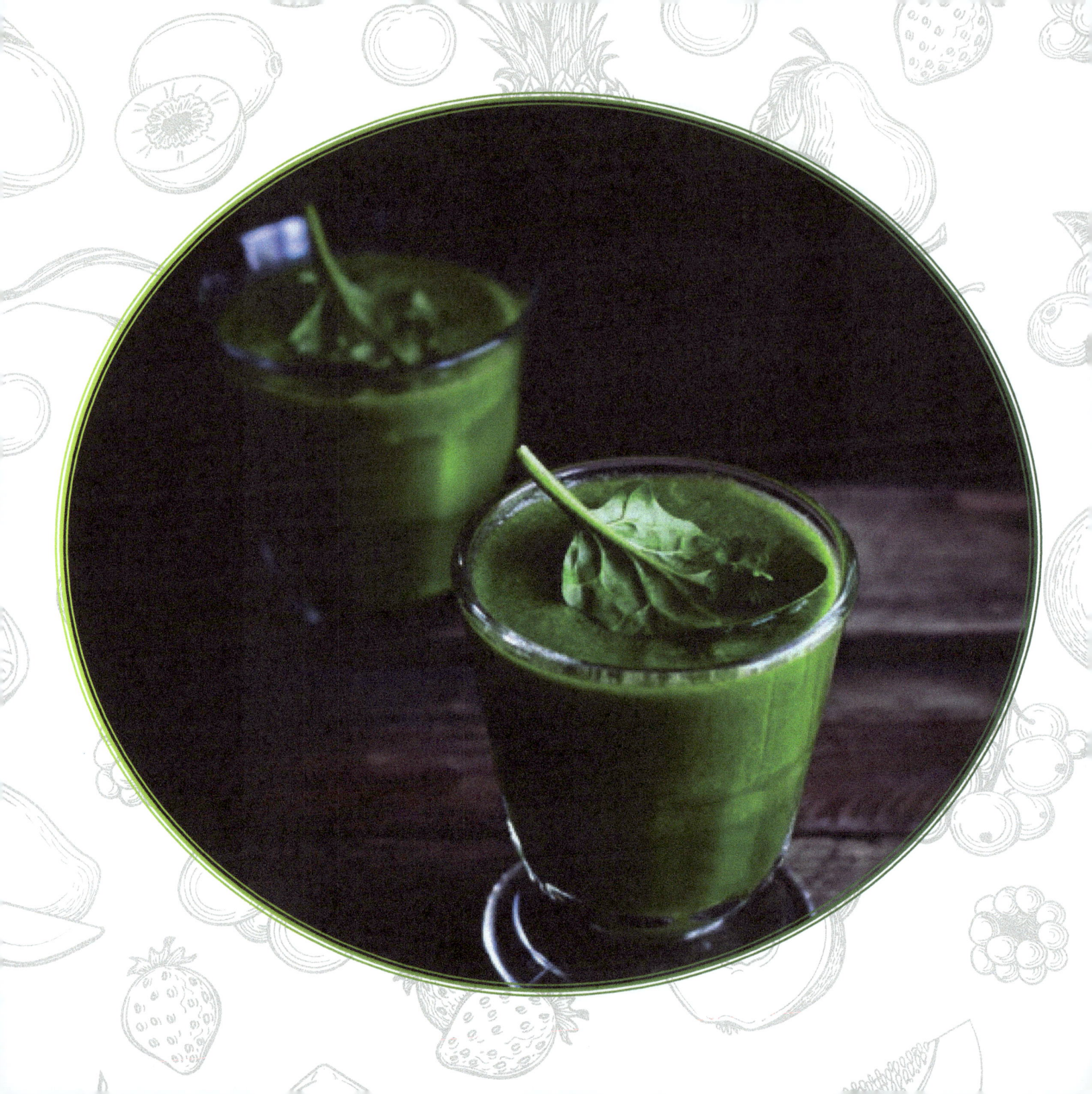

The Mean Green

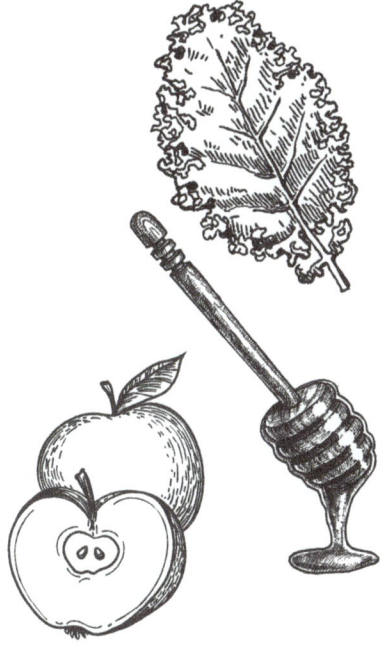

Ingredients:

1 banana

1.5 cup spinach

1.5 cup kale

3 green apples

6 ice cubes

1 cup water

1 tbsp honey

Procedure:

1) Remove peels, seeds, stems and piths from all fruit before blending.

2) Place liquid into blender (water, coconut milk, almond milk can also be used) with ice cubes. Blend till ice begins to break.

3) Add solid fruit first, blend, then add softer fruit and yoghurt if required and blend till smooth.

You are what you do, not what you say you will do.

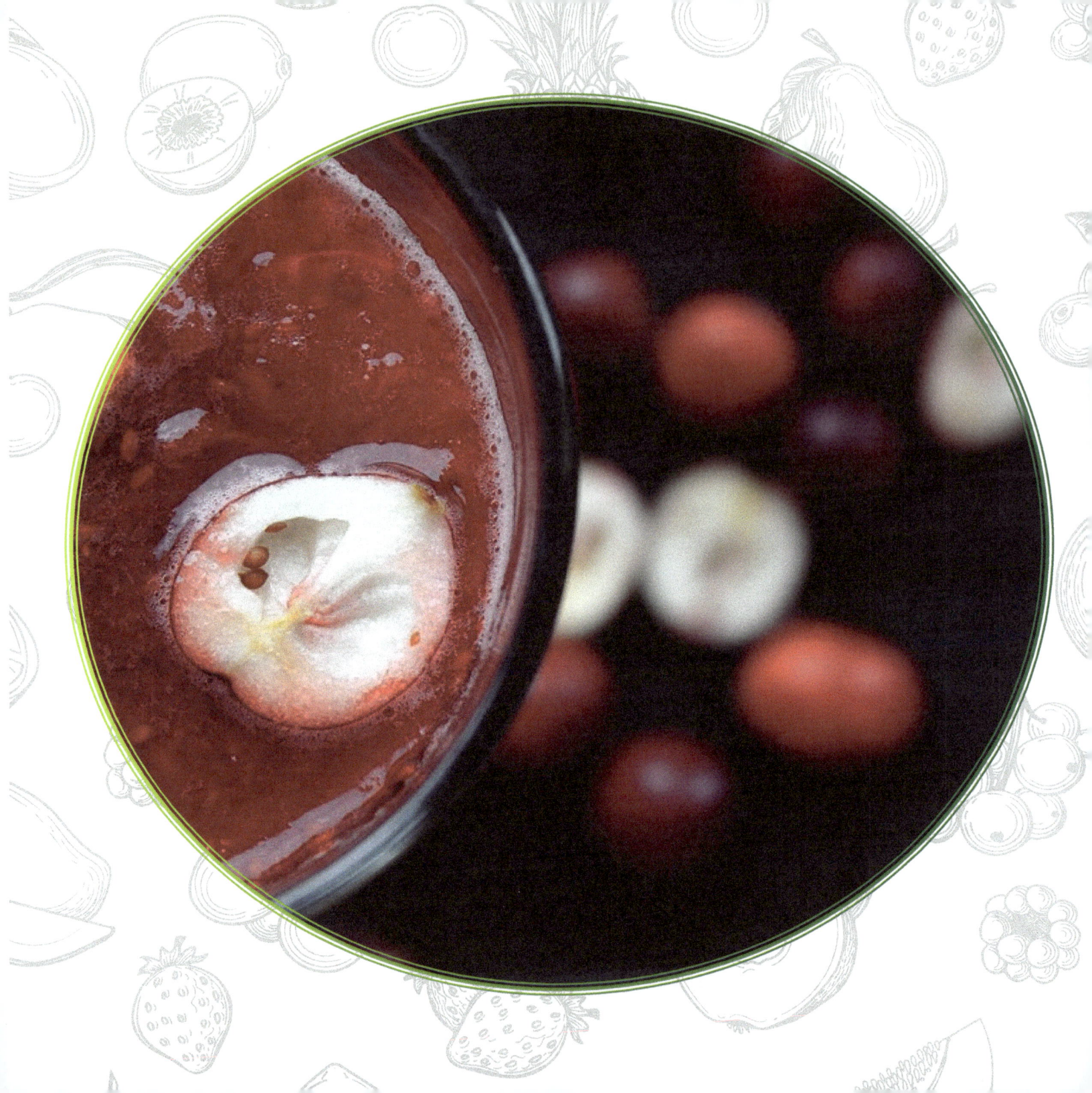

Peary Cranberry

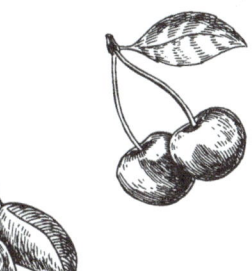

Ingredients:

1 cup cranberries

2 pears

2 apricots

1 cup cherry

½ cup coconut yoghurt

1 cup coconut milk

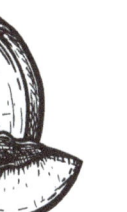

Procedure:

1) Remove peels, seeds, stems and piths from all fruit before blending.

2) Place liquid into blender (water, coconut milk, almond milk can also be used) with ice cubes. Blend till ice begins to break.

3) Add solid fruit first, blend, then add softer fruit and yoghurt if required and blend till smooth.

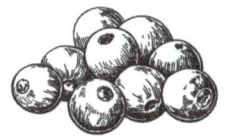

THE QUESTION IS NOT WHO'S GOING TO LET ME?
THE QUESTION IS WHO'S GOING TO STOP ME?

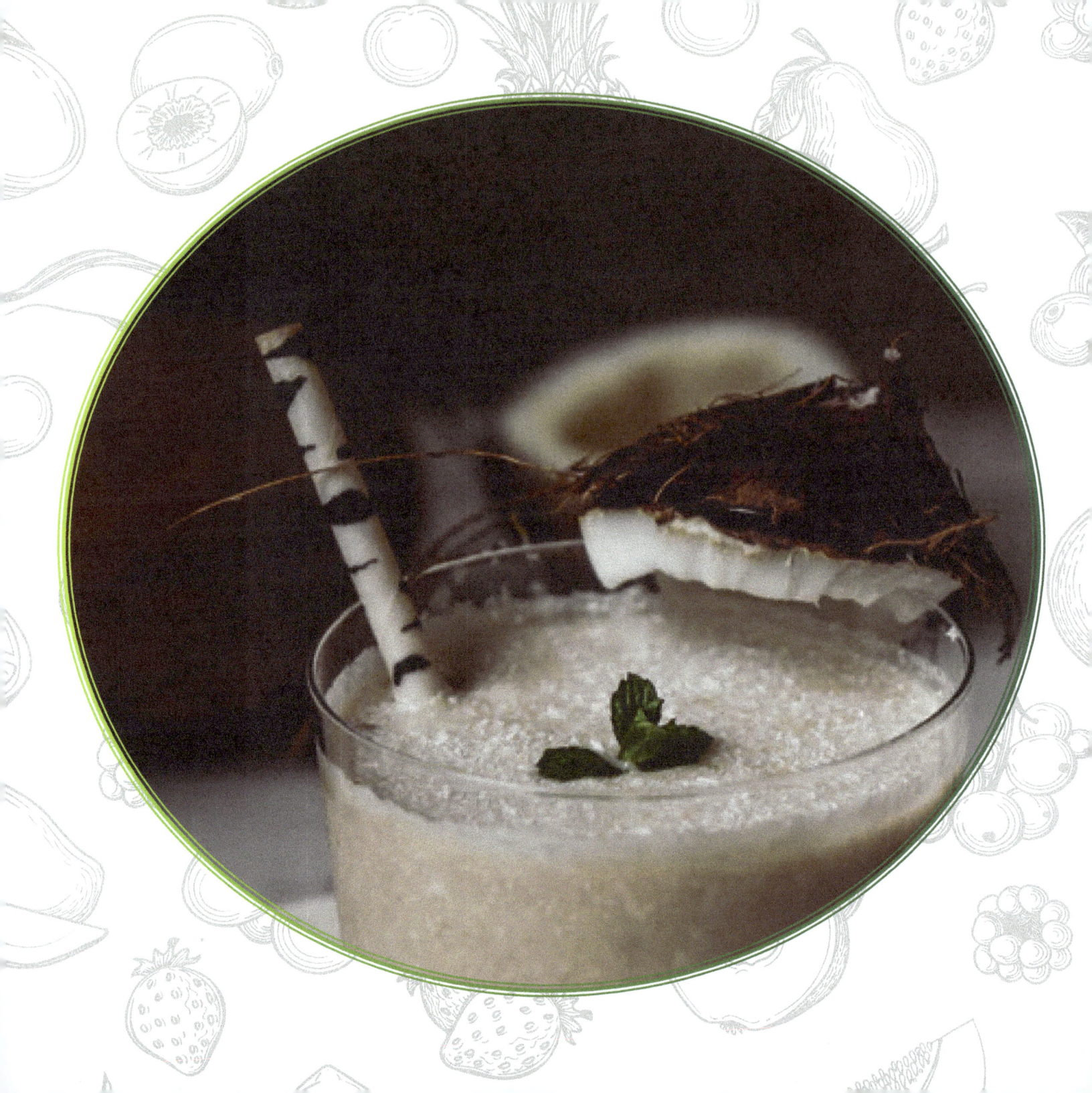

Peachy Coconut

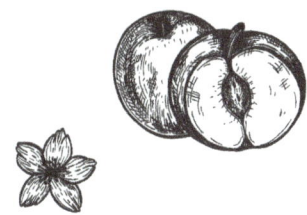

Ingredients:

3 peaches

1 cup coconut fresh

1 banana

1 cup coconut milk

½ cup coconut yoghurt

1 tsp ground flax seed

6 ice cubes

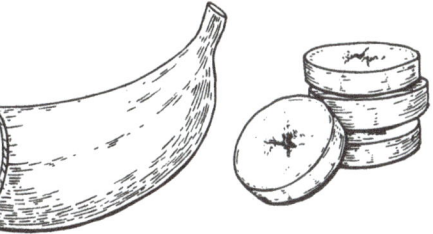

Procedure:

1) Remove peels, seeds, stems and piths from all fruit before blending.

2) Place liquid into blender (water, coconut milk, almond milk can also be used) with ice cubes. Blend till ice begins to break.

3) Add solid fruit first, blend, then add softer fruit and yoghurt if required and blend till smooth.

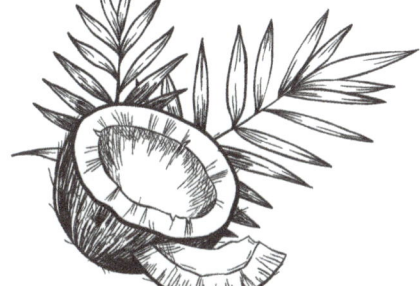

If you obey all the rules, you miss all the fun.

Lightning Source UK Ltd.
Milton Keynes UK
UKHW021334240720
367097UK00007B/97

9 780473 496531